Easy Tips for a Healthy Heart

Natural Health Series

Dueep J. Singh

Mendon Cottage Books

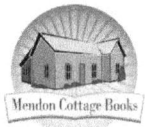

JD-Biz Publishing

Disclaimer

The information is this book is provided for informational purposes only. It is not intended to be used and medical advice or a substitute for proper medical treatment by a qualified health care provider. The information is believed to be accurate as presented based on research by the author.

The contents have not been evaluated by the U.S. Food and Drug Administration or any other Government or Health Organization and the contents in this book are not to be used to treat cure or prevent disease.

The author or publisher is not responsible for the use or safety of any diet, procedure or treatment mentioned in this book. The author or publisher is not responsible for errors or omissions that may exist.

Warning

The Book is for informational purposes only and before taking on any diet, treatment or medical procedure, it is recommended to consult with your primary health care provider.

Our books are available at

1. Amazon.com
2. Barnes and Noble
3. Itunes
4. Kobo
5. Smashwords
6. Google Play Books

Table of Contents

Introduction

Did you know that about 26.6 million people in the USA alone are suffering from heart disease? Multiply this many times, and you are going to find that heart ailments are one of the most potentially fatal diseases, all over the globe known to mankind.

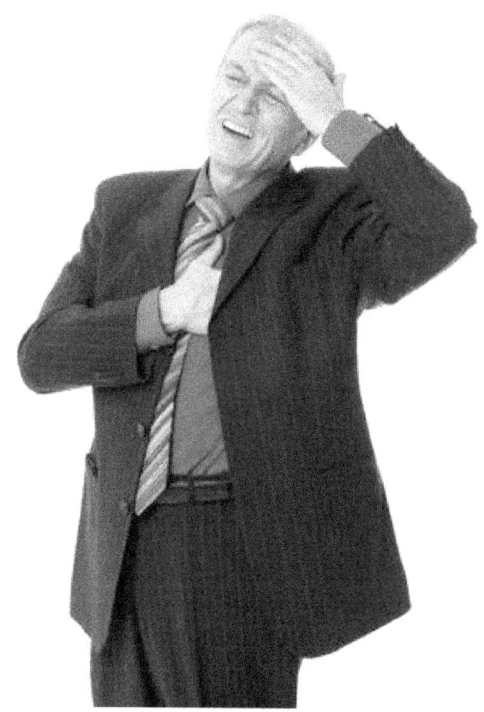

In ancient times, heart diseases were normally treated with superstitious awe. The terrible pain of a heart attack was considered to be a punishment from the gods who sent pain and split a heart and killed the wicked person. As people grew more and more sophisticated and knowledgeable, doctors began to look for ways and means in which they go to alleviate the problems of people suffering from heart disease.

Some of the remedies, especially remedies using digitalis – foxglove – could only be used by experienced wise men. Foxglove, when taken in large quantities was definitely poisonous. On the other hand, in very small quantities, it stimulated the heart, in the shape of an extract called digoxin. The use of this extract to help treat heart diseases was supposedly "discovered" in 2012 by researchers.

What they did not tell the general public was that alternative medicine practitioners all over the world have been using foxglove to treat heart diseases down the centuries. But then they knew their public. This news had to be told with lots of fanfare, publicity and statistics that a natural plant extract could help treat heart diseases before people would subject themselves to treatment by it.

This book is going to give you a lot of time-tested tips to help keep your heart healthy. All of them are common sense tips and most of them have a scientific basis.

They do not come under the alternative medicine category, because they talk about diet, stress management, exercise, and other ways in which you can keep your heart healthy. And all these factors are definitely going to be told to you by your own doctor, when you go for your normal medical checkup every three months or so.

Prevention of Heart Disease

People who are genetically prone to heart disease are going to be more vulnerable to potential heart ailments in their lifetime when compared to people who have a strong genetic background. Nevertheless, even though a person may be suffering from heart disease, with a little bit of know-how and knowledge, it is possible to control the disease from progressing further.

Dr. Dean Ornish brought this concept to the notice of Americans in the early 70s. But then he was already bringing the scientific equivalent of "the Wisdom of the Ages" into view.

The lifestyle plan, which has been suggested by Dr. Ornish has been followed for millenniums by millions of people, and it was only after Medicare decided to support his findings and programs that more and more people began to think that there was something in what he said!

Well, friends, I looked through the program and I was surprised to see that this program consisted of meditation, vegetarian diet, aerobic exercise, breathing exercises, stress management and other tips and techniques, and so on – all of which came under the heading of "a lifestyle practice by the ancients millenniums ago."

So even if it is old wine in a new bottle, anything that keeps you healthy is all to the good. Dr. Ornish's results are now widely accepted all over the world. His programs include a modification of your lifestyle, evaluation of the risk factors which cause a disease, or which can prevent this disease from occurring, stress management, meditation, yoga, proper diet, counseling, cessation of alcohol and tobacco abuse, and exercise prescriptions based on the functional capacity of an individual.

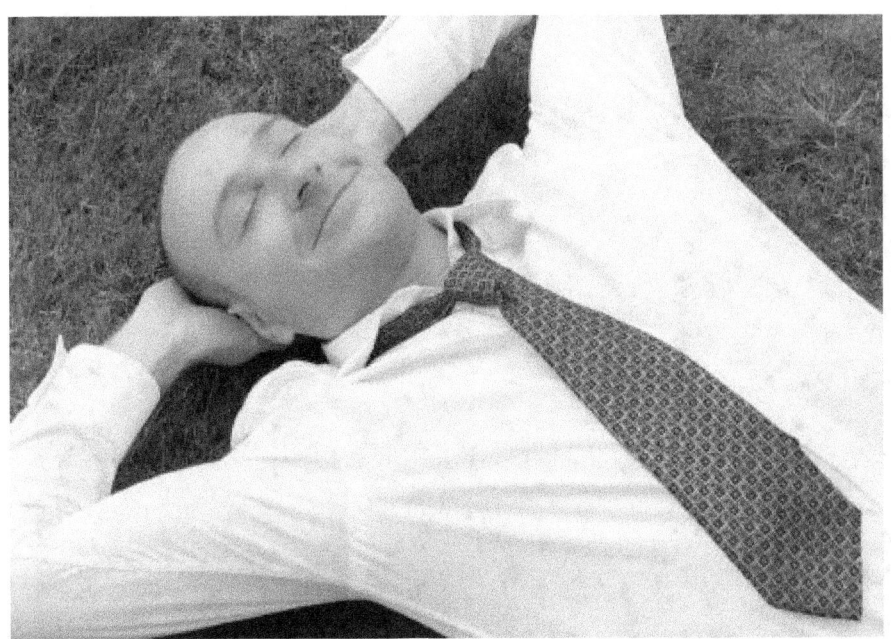

We are slowly forgetting the art of relaxation without stress and tension, in this day and age.

The greatest universal truths are the simplest ones. But it takes a little while for man to acknowledge the wisdom of what is being told to him. Dr. Dean Ornish was not taken seriously at all, in the beginning of his research because his experienced colleagues considered himself to be too young, too inexperienced and too radical. That was because they were not willing to listen to anything which was a drastic change from their own concept of medical knowledge and learned theories.

Cholesterol

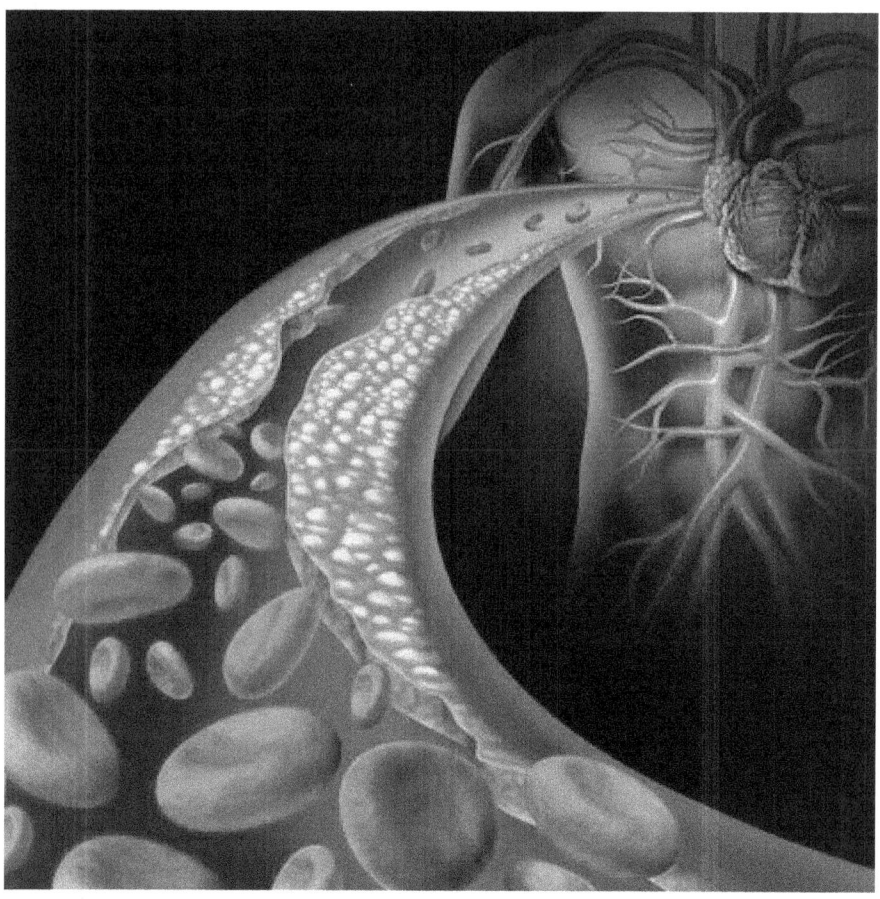

One of the main important risk factors causing heart disease on which Dr. Ornish concentrated was cholesterol. Many of us have heard about cholesterol, but we do not know about its importance. The presence or absence of cholesterol in our body is going to make all the difference between a healthy heart, or an ailing one.

There are certain conditions, and lifestyles which are now universally recognized and documented to be responsible at the deposition of cholesterol and fat in your blood vessels. The main cause of a Coronary Heart Disease – C HD – or a Coronary Artery Disease – CAD – or Ischemic Heart Disease – IHD – is the deposition of fat and cholesterol in the indoor smooth lining of your coronary arteries. These are the blood vessels which supply blood to the heart.

This plaque deposition results in blockages and obstruction of your blood flow through these arteries. A high blood cholesterol level is considered to be one of the well-known factors which can contribute to heart disease.

What Is Cholesterol?

Cholesterol is a type of fat particle which is present in the blood in small quantities. It is waxy in constitution, and is made up of a single chain of fatty acids, with 27 carbon atoms. This is one of the most complex fatty acids structures known to chemists, and that is the reason why they have given it a long scary name called a cyclo–pentane-perhydro-phenantherene ring.

Well, the name can be justified, because this cholesterol has a very important part to play in the functioning of the body. It forms a major part of the cell wall, the coverings of the nerves and the brain cells. It is so important in the normal functioning of a living being's system that the liver needs required quantity of cholesterol every day in order to keep your system moving smoothly and in a healthy fashion.

However, if this particular molecule is present in more quantities than what is required in your blood or in your body, the excess accumulation of this fatty acid is going to be deposited in your arteries. This means that it is going to create some blockages, which are called coronary blockages.

That means the normal blood supply to your brain and to your heart is going to be affected. Apart from this, high cholesterol levels, blocking your arteries are going to affect your leg arteries, the skin below the eyes, and also the arteries inside the brain.

Any person who is not a science student, or even a chemist can thus easily understand that this deposit is potentially dangerous.

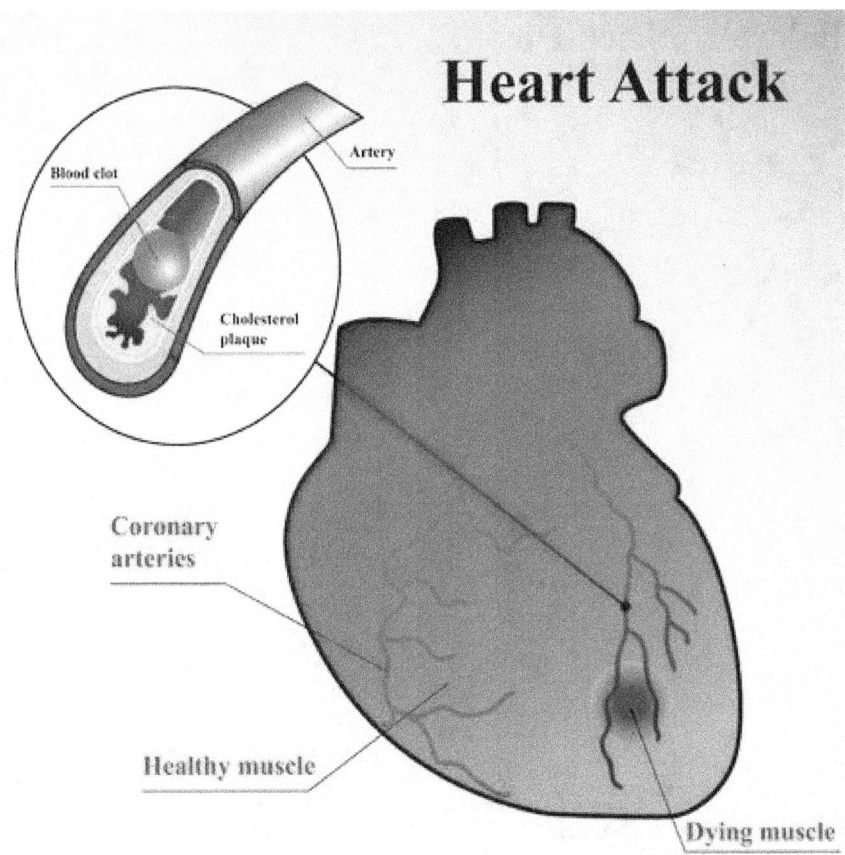

This cholesterol is carried in the blood in a free form. When it mixes up with lipoproteins, which are very common in fatty and protein rich food items, you can considered this combination to be as potentially lethal as dynamite.

So if you have a high level of free cholesterol in your blood, the chances of you suffering from a blockage in your arteries grow proportionately.

Cholesterol Rich Diet

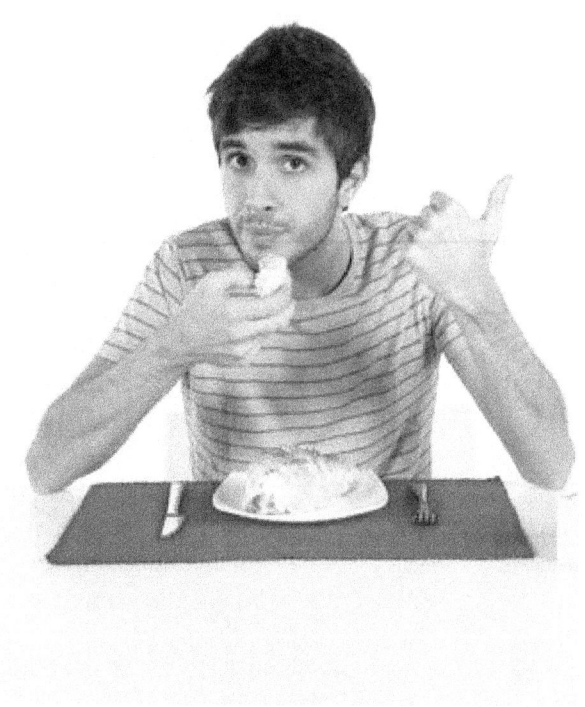

Creamy cake now means heart and cholesterol problems tomorrow...

The blood levels of cholesterol are going to be very high in those people who like eating a diet rich in cholesterol. These foods include egg yolk, meat, mutton, beef, chicken, pork, and fish. Another resource of cholesterol is milk and all its products like cream, butter, clarified butter, ice cream, yogurt and cottage cheese.

This dependence on milk products is the reason why so many vegetarians find themselves suffering from high cholesterol. That is because they are depending upon milk to give them the necessary proteins and nutrients in order to keep healthy.

Any other fat, especially the oils which we use for deep frying our food – whether they have an animal or a vegetable base – especially saturated fatty acids, are used in the liver to manufacture cholesterol.

Is a Zero Fat Diet Beneficial?

Just go onto the Internet, and do a Google search on zero fat diet. You are going to be surprised to see the amount of supposedly serious weight loss gurus and health gurus recommending zero fat. They know not of what they speak. Man cannot do without fat.

Like I told you before, our bodies need a little bit of cholesterol in order to keep functioning properly. That is the reason why a totally zero fat diet is harmful, even though many dietitians consider this to be good for your health. It is not – you need some fat to keep your liver functioning properly.

However, a fat intake should be regulated in such a manner that your liver does not manufacture excess of cholesterol. So there is no chance of any cholesterol deposit.

Triglycerides

Apart from cholesterol, triglycerides are the other fats, which have gained importance in the latest series of research studies to prevent and control heart disease. These are also major factors which contribute to heart ailments. Oils contain lots of triglycerides.

All kinds of oil is going to be hundred percent fat, irrespective of any combination of saturated, mono unsaturated and poly saturated percentages being marketed by unscrupulous and unethical companies.

Triglycerides are definitely not good for your heart, whatever the advertising may say. So if you hear about an oil which supposedly helps in curing heart disease in heart patients, being marketed extensively, take these words as blatant lies, and with a huge pinch of salt.

High Blood Pressure

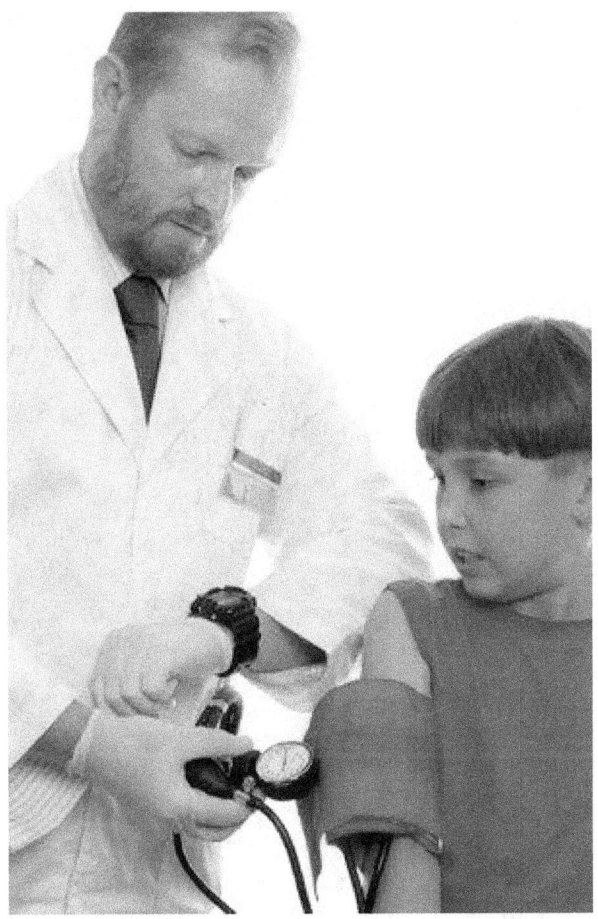

A normal blood pressure in adults is between 100/60 – 140/90 mm Hg. If your blood pressure is consistently more than 140/90 on more than two separate occasions, your doctor is going to tell you that you are suffering from hypertension, also known as High Blood Pressure.

Main complications of hypertension

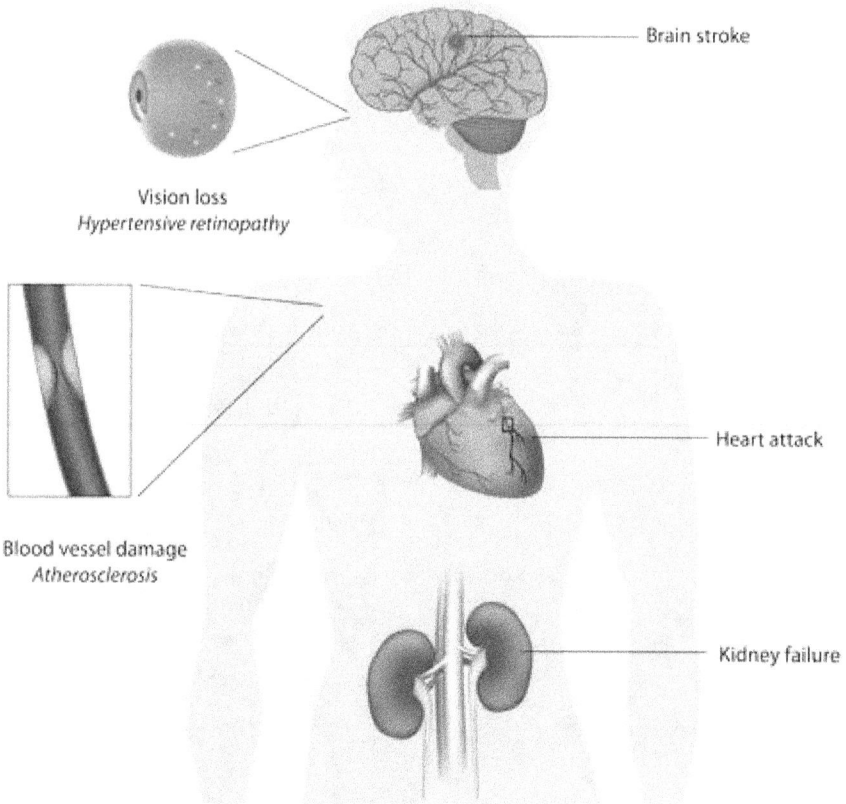

This is a very common disease and about 30% of adults suffer from hypertension, all over the world. You are going to be surprised to know that many of them do not know that they are suffering from the silent killer, because according to them, they are not showing any symptoms, which tells them that stress, strain, a high intake of salt, etc. has given rise to hypertension in them.

High blood pressure is going to put an extra strain on your heart as well as on the arteries which supply blood to the other organs of your body. This is the major factor in causing other ailments like kidney failure, heart attacks, heart failure, strokes and other related ailments.

High blood pressure is one of the main reasons why cholesterol gets deposited in your coronary arteries. That is because it is damages the inner lining of your arteries, making them more prone to a deposit of fat.

How does that happen? Let me explain – Just imagine blood being pumped at a high pressure through a particular artery. This pressure rubs away the lining of the artery. That area can now be covered by a layer of cholesterol, where once there were cells. So this artery is now prone to cholesterol blockage.

Diabetes and Coronary Blockages

A normal level of blood sugar in a fasting person should be between 80 – 120 mg %.

If your fasting level of blood sugar is more than 110 mg % and after meals, it is more than 160 mg it is called high blood sugar, or Diabetes Mellitus.

Diabetic patients show sugar levels in the urine too. These patients have a higher chance of coronary blockages, because many of these patients are usually obese, have high blood pressure and high blood cholesterol levels, which are all responsible for blockages.

The symptoms of diabetes is increased thirst, increased urination and weight loss, but in some cases there may not be any symptoms at all.

Obesity – Leading to Heart Problems

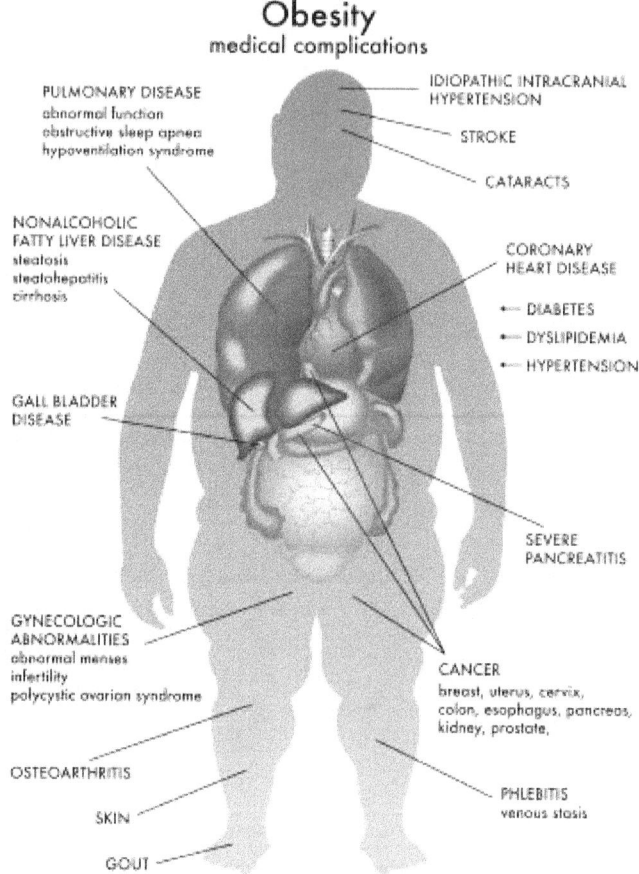

Obesity
medical complications

PULMONARY DISEASE
abnormal function
obstructive sleep apnea
hypoventilation syndrome

IDIOPATHIC INTRACRANIAL
HYPERTENSION

STROKE

CATARACTS

NONALCOHOLIC
FATTY LIVER DISEASE
steatosis
steatohepatitis
cirrhosis

CORONARY
HEART DISEASE

DIABETES

DYSLIPIDEMIA

HYPERTENSION

GALL BLADDER
DISEASE

SEVERE
PANCREATITIS

GYNECOLOGIC
ABNORMALITIES
abnormal menses
infertility
polycystic ovarian syndrome

CANCER
breast, uterus, cervix,
colon, esophagus, pancreas,
kidney, prostate,

OSTEOARTHRITIS

SKIN

PHLEBITIS
venous stasis

GOUT

If the weight of a person is more than the upper limit of weight for that age group, and gender, he is called an obese or a fat person. People who eat too much fat and do not exercise start to put on weight.

There are plenty of standard charts available from which one can find out whether one is overweight or obese.

http://www.dietbites.com/article1023.html

This is not to be used as a medical guide, but just for general reference.

Obese individuals have greater chances of getting heart diseases. They also have increased chances of high blood pressure and diabetes, including blockages.

Obesity can be prevented by eating low-calorie food, avoiding fats, avoiding too much sugar and also exercising regularly.

Fat people normally have a sedentary lifestyle. They become lethargic because it is difficult for them to move about in an agile fashion, which they did when they were slimmer. So they remain sedentary. This lack of exercise causes them to grow even more bulky and fat. This then is a vicious circle, because the fatter you are, the more you are not going to be inclined to do any sort of exercise.

Such people are going to develop some sort of mental tension, because they consider themselves to be physically unattractive. They know that they are fat, but they are not willing to take steps to counteract the state, either through a proper regulated diet or through some sort of physical exercise. They would rather sit and say self pityingly, "I am really so bad, I do not know what I am going to do about that," with one hand reaching out towards a cream filled chocolate éclair.

This lack of exercise, and regulated diet, stress and tension is going to result in hypertension and an increased chance of a heart attack. The chances of obese people getting heart attacks is 15% more than that of a thin person.

Dieting to Reduce Obesity

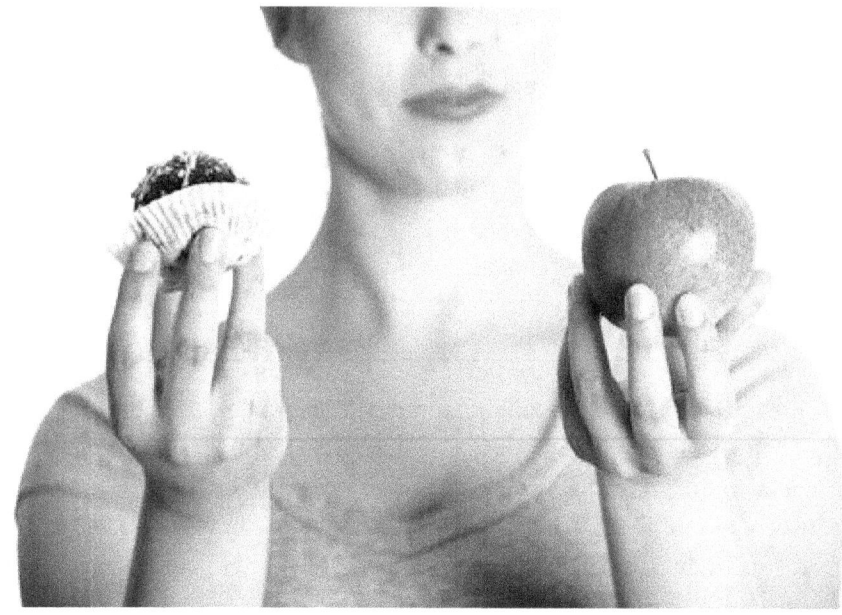

Did you know that a number of people who find themselves gaining weight, and are on the borderline to obesity, suddenly decide that they need to go on a drastic diet. This is the only way in which they can get rid of all that accumulated fatty tissue. So they immediately start to starve themselves.

Now for anybody who is thinking of going on a strict dieting regime or program so that he can lose weight really fast, he needs to look at two things.

Ask your medical caretaker about whether he advises you to go on your diet. He is going to take your state of health in view, and then give you the go-ahead signal or possibly he is going to say no, you are in no condition to starve yourself. Do not do it.

Many of the diets which are being endorsed by rock stars and superstars on different media channels are not going to tell you all about the harmful side effects. You may find yourself really amazed, because you lost weight in supposedly 48 hours. This whole program is definitely going to be detrimental to the state of your health, because it just got rid of all the extra toxins built up in your body.

You are really glad, because according to you, you have lost weight. You have not lost weight – you are just got rid of all the extra fluids. They are going to get accumulated again in the next two – three months.

A good diet loss program should not be more than 48 hours at the most. If you find yourself starving yourself of all the essential nutrients which you need to keep yourself healthy, your body is going to be deprived of all these important minerals in the future, and thus suffer accordingly.

Any sort of reduction diet should just get rid of two – 3 pounds in one month.

Crash diets are not recommended. Systematic diets should be those types of diets which do not permit you to starve yourself. If you think that skipping meals is going to make you healthy, because after all, you are not eating something and there is no question of you getting fat, you are mistaken.

You are soon going to reach the stage when your body begins to suffer from malnutrition. It knows that it is not getting the necessary nutrients. So it will begin to store fat because it knows that without this fat, all your organs are going to slow down and soon they will begin to fail.

So, never skip meals.

Medical Tests

There are a number of tests, available for the confirmation of any sort of coronary heart disease.

A physical checkup is done before any other tests are ordered by your medical practitioner. This is a complete physical examination of the patient, including the measurement of blood pressure and pulse rate. A lipid profile as well as blood sugar tests are also going to be taken by the clinic.

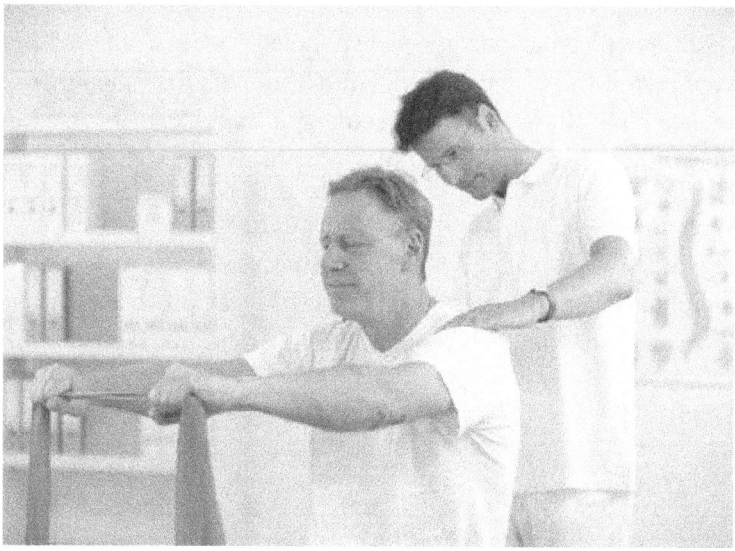

After that, your cardiologist may recommend an electrocardiogram, or **ECG** test. If your electrocardiogram does not provide any conclusive evidence of a heart disease, you may be asked to do a treadmill test – **TMT** – test.

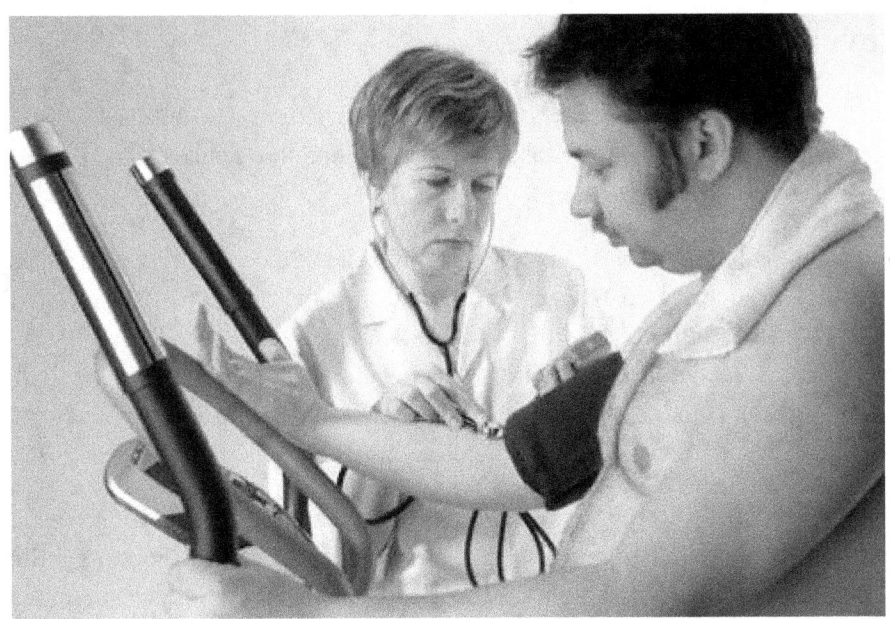

This treadmill test is recommended to only those people who are physically fit enough to bear the physical stress of walking on a treadmill. This test, along with an ECG test is considered to be a safe and noninvasive test for the confirmation of any sort of CAD.

A cardiogram – **ECHO** – is done to find out all about the pumping power of your heart. It is also going to give your cardiologist reliable information about the condition of the heart walls.

Angiography – I consider this to be a rather futile test, because it is costly, imprecise, and it also carries a definite risk in itself. Here, a long wire is going to fill blocked tubes of the heart with an opaque dye, which can be monitored on a screen. Afterwards, you are going to get an approximate percentage of the blockages.

Those people to whom cardiologists have recommended a bypass surgery or even an angioplasty should go in for angiography. But seriously speaking, bypass surgeries and angioplasty are fast becoming the rule instead of the exception for a number of cardiologists, who would rather have their patients shell out lots of money in getting these expensive operations done.

They do not tell them that it is possible to reverse heart disease.

Reversing Heart Disease

Is it really possible to reverse heart disease? Well, believe it or not, in most cases, people suffering from heart diseases have been cured through rigorous discipline, diet

Being an ex-administrator of a cardiac hospital and having met a number of these patients, I was surprised when they used to ask me, "ma'am, I went to ABC cardiac hospital, and they said that I needed a bypass. And here I have been told that it is easy for a heart disease to be reversed. I do not need this bypass operation done. Is that true? "And then they would be surprised when I said "you have been tested. Your coronary blockage can and will be reversed. You will be cured."

This is not a miracle. It is proven fact . In 90% of the cases, the most rational solution to a coronary heart disease is going to lie in the permanent process, which not only arrest the progress of the blockage *but also reverses the same.*

Let me admit in all truth. In 85% of the cases, the patients visiting our hospital did not need an angioplasty or a bypass done. But other unscrupulous doctors in other cardio hospitals had immediately scared them so much that they had immediately got these expensive operations done. And they were reassured that their life spans were increased, because of the experience of Dr. ABC who is well-known for doing so many successful bypass surgeries.

Dr. ABC is a multimillionaire. He has gained his millions by scaring his patients who trust him. There are plenty of Dr. ABCs in your own city. So rather than get into his clutches, and go through a traumatic surgical process,

So once you know after a checkup that there is some sort of blockage in your arteries, this is what really happened.

This blockage has occurred over a given period of time, consisting of several years. That was because the cholesterol from the blood flowed through the coronary arteries and got deposited in the arterial wall.

These deposits are mostly soft masses of fat with connective tissues. *They happen to be in a reversible phase.*

It has scientifically been proven that cholesterol and fat can dissolve in blood and they can be picked up from the blockages, if you can create an ideal situation for this process to occur.

This is why in ancient times, people who suffer from obesity were immediately put under a strict regime. That was to melt off all the fat literally from their bodies. They were not allowed to smoke or to drink. They were given vegetarian food to eat, rich in organic fruit and vegetables.

Remember that any sort of reversible heart disease regime is not magic. If you expect all that accumulated fat of the ages to get removed in the next 21 days, right in time for you to wow them at your cousin's wedding, sorry, no can do.

However, if the wedding is going to take place in six month's time, you can start on this health improvement magic right now.

It is going to take at least two weeks to see the first sign of improvement. This improvement is going to depend on the effort put in by the patient, his age, the stage of blockage, the support and the cooperation of family members and other factors like self-discipline and strict diet.

Remember that they are plenty of books which can give you information on heart disease reversal processes. But all this theoretical knowledge is of no use unless it is backed up with practical knowledge.

So as long as you know how to translate that knowledge into a practical and physical form, you are not going to get any benefit from the written word.

Here are some lifestyle changes, which you can practice right now –

Your exercise routine which includes yoga, meditation, and light physical labor should not be more than about an hour a day. Do lots of walking. Meditation means sitting in a calm and tranquil atmosphere and trying to relax. This is an excellent stress buster. Unfortunately, most of us are so busy in the rat race of getting ahead of the Joneses that we forget to relax and even do a little bit of deep breathing of fresh oxygen.

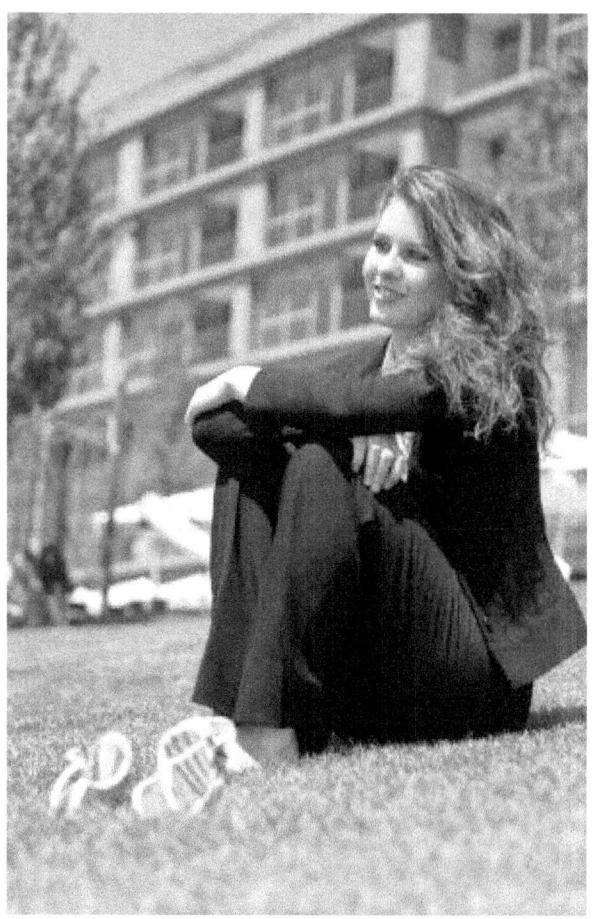

How often have you done this in the past couple of months?

Smoking and tobacco abuse is a definite no-no. In the same way, a strictly vegetarian diet is the best way in which you can keep your heart healthy.

Rational Treatment Regime

Your goal is to control or modify the risk factors for the development of heart disease.

Physically, you are going to develop a regular physical activity and exercise regimen. You are also going to maintain a normal body weight.

Medically, you aim to maintain a normal blood pressure, normal serum cholesterol, normal HDL-cholesterol, normal blood sugar and normal serum triglycerides.

Your behavioral factors are going to include proper management of anxiety, stress, anger and worry. You are also going to say an absolute no to any tobacco-related products, including snuff and smokes. Milk products, especially fatty milk, butter and cream is strictly taboo. Your oil intake is going to be limited. Also, highly proteinaceous food like meat, fish and eggs are going to be removed from your diet.

How Much Physical Activity Do You Need to Do?

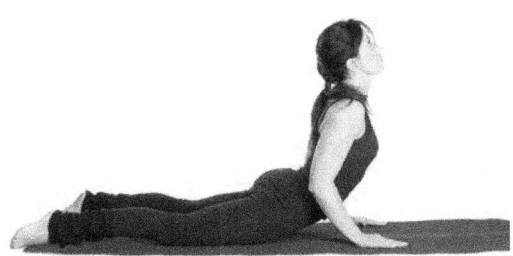

This is going to depend on your age, the state of your health, and your level of physical fitness. If you are 60 years old, and are suffering from heart disease, asking you to climb up the three flights of stairs three times a day is very foolish. On the other hand, your doctor is going to suggest that you do a little bit of regular walking, morning and evening, to get your system working properly.

This exercise regime means that all the collaterals in your circulatory system – the small tubes which are closed and which take over the functions once the normal arteries of the heart gets clogged – open up. That means your circulatory system is waking up and healing itself.

Your Dietary Habits –

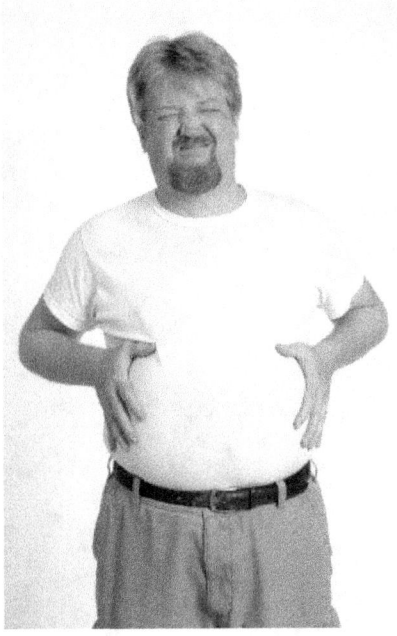

CAD normally occurs because of the development of blockages due to the deposits of cholesterol and triglycerides present in your arteries. Unless and until you stop the supply of fats and oils from outside, you cannot get rid of the disease.

Hence, the food that you eat should be totally free of fat and oil, except for the amount told to you by your doctor to keep your kidneys functioning properly.

Milk which is an animal product should be stopped. However, you may want to substitute soy bean milk on the advice of your doctor. This is healthier.

Vegetarian food, which is full of antioxidants and fiber should be added to your diet right now.

Yoga and Meditation

What is Yoga?

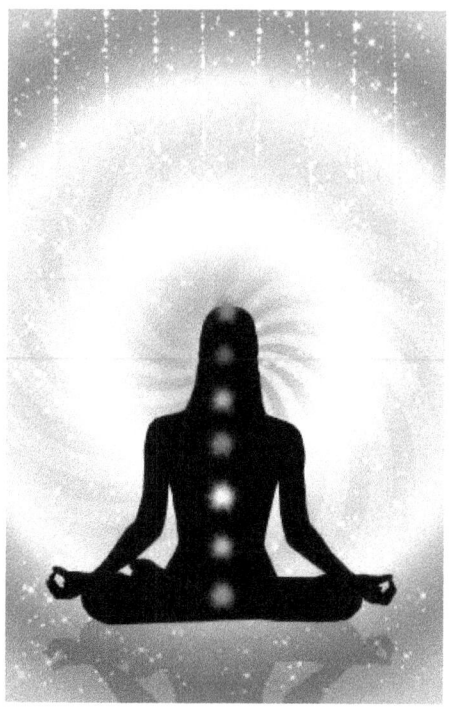

Yoga is a philosophical doctrine, which developed in the Indian subcontinent about 4 – 5000 years ago. It was based on meditational techniques, moral principles and also on exercises, postures and respiration. In the same manner, similar doctrines were developing in China and in other parts of Asia and the Orient based on the same principles. These doctrines are still being used in the East to keep one mentally, emotionally, spiritually, physically, and psychologically fit.

Yoga and relaxation have been successfully used for the amelioration of high blood pressure and coronary heart diseases for a number of years in the West. Recent researches have proven that this form of treatment not only reduces high blood pressure, but it also reduces the serum cholesterol levels, serum triglyceride levels, serum free fatty acid, blood glucose, body weight and CAD.

Unlike medical drugs, this form of therapy has absolutely no side effects. Continuous UV practice also improves your physical fitness and helps to improve your energy levels.

I am still surprised when people come to me and tell me that they do not bother much about yoga, because after all, it is more of an ancient esoteric Eastern tantra mantra. I would beg to differ.

Yoga is definitely not related to religion. It is a way of life. It came into existence millenniums ago, when religions did not play such a major role in the social fabric. Nevertheless, down the ages wise men decided that the only way in which they could get their acolytes, and people of the tribe to practice these exercises and keep healthy, was to get them to chant some mantras and chants.

Thus yogic exercises got related to chants. All over the East, people of other religions also followed physical exercises with spiritual chants. In this way they were doing two things at one time. They were gaining good karma by meditating and praying. At the same time, their bodies were going through a proper physical workout.

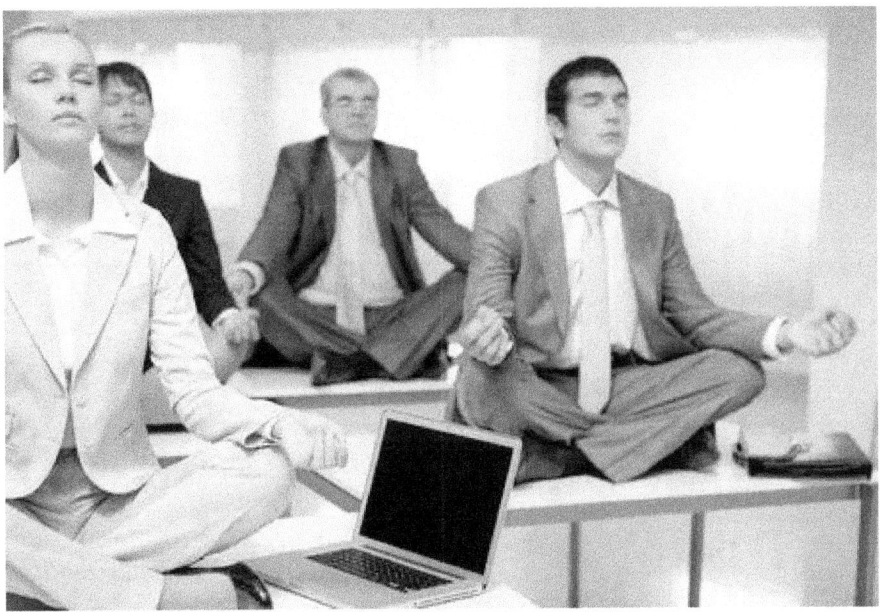

So remember that yoga is nondenominational. It belongs to mankind. It is not the exclusive property of one caste, religion, creed, race, or denomination. In the same way, meditation does not mean that you have to chant a given chant. You can say whatever you want.

For example, I take about 20 minutes out of a busy schedule to sit cross legged on the ground or even on the sofa. I need a little bit of stress busting. I switch on my Walkman and wait for whatever comes through the system.

It might be a Gregorian chant, which I downloaded at http://inchoro.net/ , it may be Buddham Sharanam gacchami or Om Name padme hum, or Om or the Mool Mantar, whatever switches on is going to give me spiritual strength. This was the way in which the ancients got people to do physical exercises, by getting them to do prayers.So I, being born a human being, pray my own way while meditating, and thus get rid of stress and strain.

Believe it or not, faith has a lot to do with helping cure you.

How to Practice Yoga

You can meditate for as long as you want. The best time to practice yoga and relaxation is early in the morning, which is very convenient for all of us who need to get to the office every day.

Make sure that you do yoga on an empty stomach. Do not eat before or after this routine. Put on clothes which are loose fitting. Your surroundings should be quiet. You can do your routine in a well ventilated room, or in the open air.

Remember that you need to do these routines regularly. It is of no use if you do yoga exercises for 10 days in the initial burst of enthusiasm and suddenly find that you are too tired today, so let us skip it. You are going to do the skipping tomorrow too. By day after tomorrow you will have persuaded yourself that, as you have not seen any visible improvement in 10 days, what is the use. So let us forget about it, shall we,hmmmm?

You can also do your exercises in the evening, but make sure that you have a two-hour gap before you eat your meals and do your exercises. If you need a cup of tea or milk, drink it half an hour before you start on your exercise routine.

People are very surprised when I tell them that I never got into the habit of drinking tea and coffee. [just decided as a child that these silly stimulants were not for me and stuck to it.] I believe that is the reason why I have never suffered from caffeine addiction, stress, tension, and other caffeine, tannin related problems. Also not having alcohol or nicotine ever [except a glass of champagne on my 21st birthday! Even that was vinegary. Or perhaps, it is my deplorable palate, which deemed it so.] means a clear skin, no wrinkles, no health problems, no stress, no tension, no heart problems, no diabetes, and definitely no obesity.

So along with yoga, you need 6 to 8 hours of sleep. If you go to bed early, it is going to be possible for you to wake up early in the morning to do your exercises. Then and only then it is possible to you to maintain a proper and healthy routine, including yoga practice.

While doing your yoga asanas, take rest immediately if you feel tired. Never cross the limits of your capacity. This capacity is going to increase slowly, as your body gets used to this exercise routine. Relax after you have done your exercises.

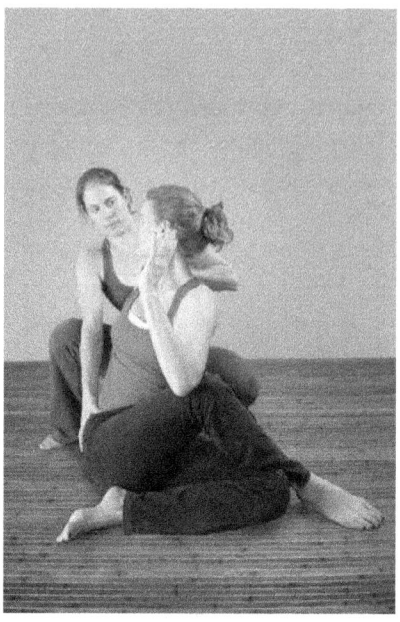

You may want to do these exercises under the guidance of a proper yoga teacher. These exercises are going to consist of relaxing exercises, breathing exercises or **pranayama,** and then kayutsarga or relaxation exercise.

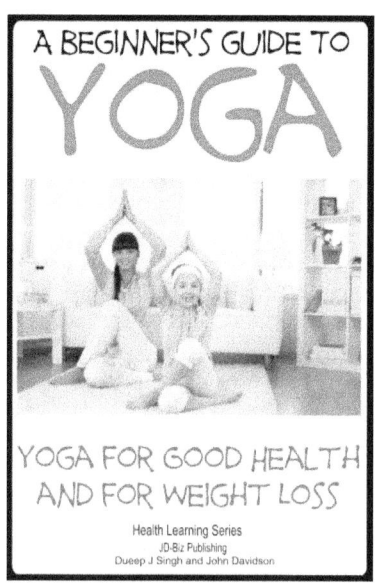

Conclusion

This book has given you lots of information on how to keep your heart healthy. You have also gained knowledge on ways in which you can reverse or prevent heart disease.

Remember many of the diseases which are being incurred by human beings in the 21st century are because of a changing lifestyle full of an uncontrolled diet and the lessening of proper physical activity. So if you do want to Live Long and Prosper, go through these easy to implement tips and May the Powers Go with You!

These are some books which are associated to heart disease. –

Health Learning Series

Author Bio-

Dueep Jyot Singh is a Management and IT Professional who managed to gather Postgraduate qualifications in Management and English and Degrees in Science, French and Education while pursuing different enjoyable career options like being a Cardiac hospital administrator, IT,SEO and HRD Database Manager/ trainer, movie , radio and TV scriptwriter, theatre artiste and public speaker, lecturer in French, Marketing and Advertising, ex-Editor of Hearts On Fire (now known as Solstice) Books Missouri USA, advice columnist and cartoonist, publisher and Aviation School trainer, ex- moderator on Medico.in, banker, student councilor ,travelogue writer … among other things!

One fine morning, she decided that she had enough of killing herself by Degrees and went back to her first love -- writing. It's more enjoyable! She already has 48 published academic and 14 fiction- in- different- genre books under her belt.

When she is not designing websites or making Graphic design illustrations for clients , she is browsing through old bookshops hunting for treasures, of which she has an enviable collection – including R.L. Stevenson, O.Henry, Dornford Yates, Maurice Walsh, De Maupassant, Victor Hugo, Sapper, C.N. Williamson, "Bartimeus" and the crown of her collection- Dickens "The Old Curiosity Shop," and so on… Just call her "Renaissance Woman") - collecting herbal remedies, acting like Universal Helping Hand/Agony Aunt, or escaping to her dear mountains for a bit of exploring, collecting herbs and plants and trekking.

Our books are available at

1. Amazon.com
2. Barnes and Noble
3. Itunes
4. Kobo
5. Smashwords
6. Google Play Books

Check out some of the other JD-Biz Publishing books
Gardening Series on Amazon

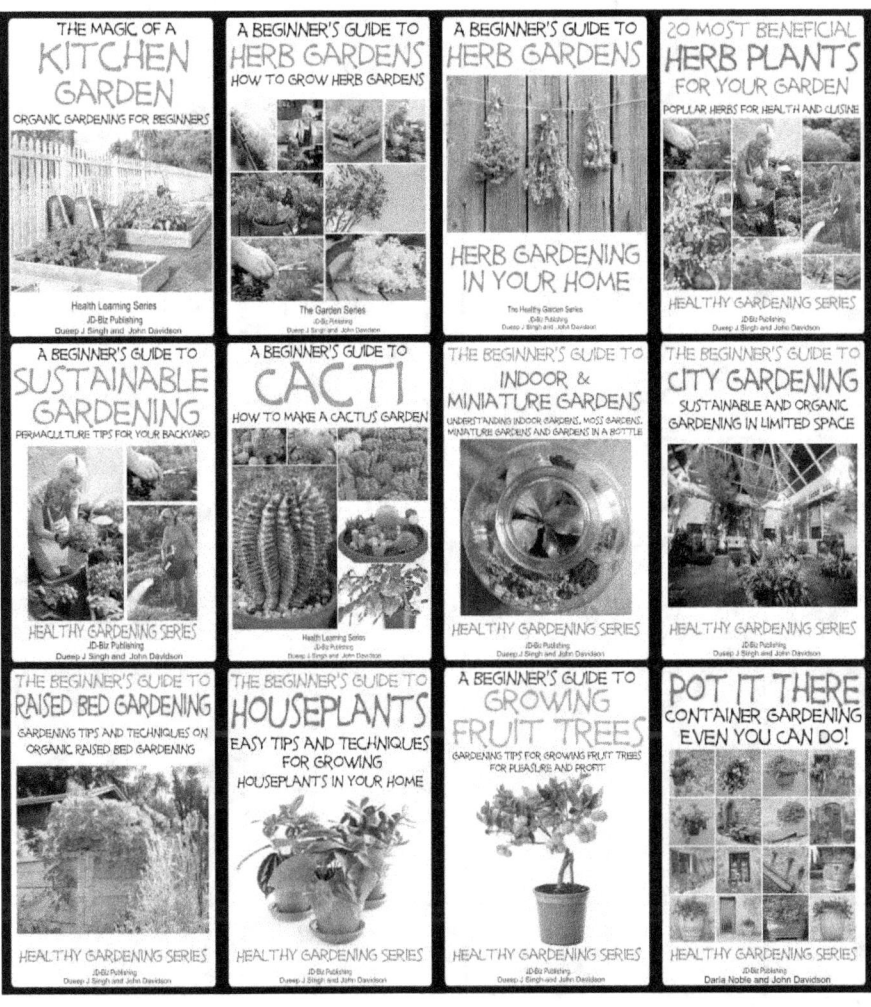

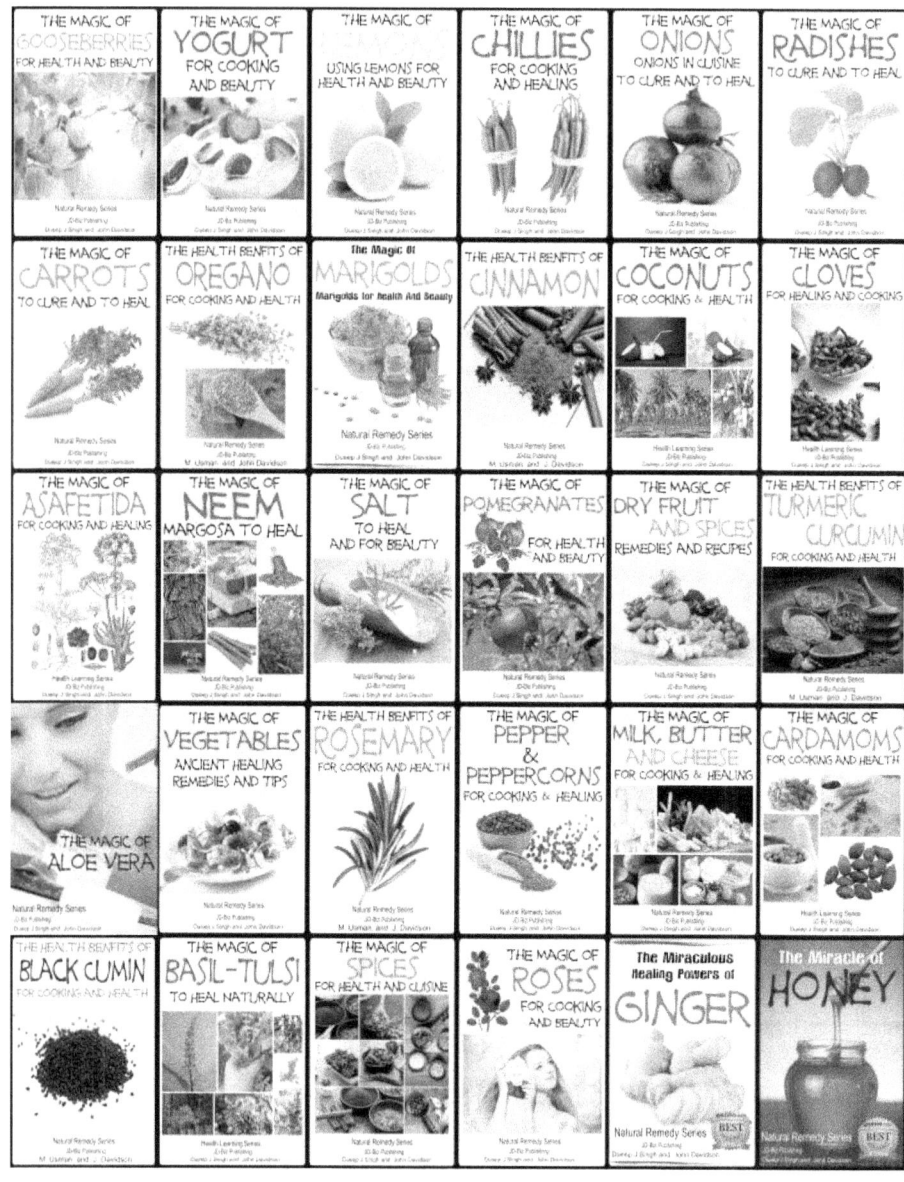

Country Life Books

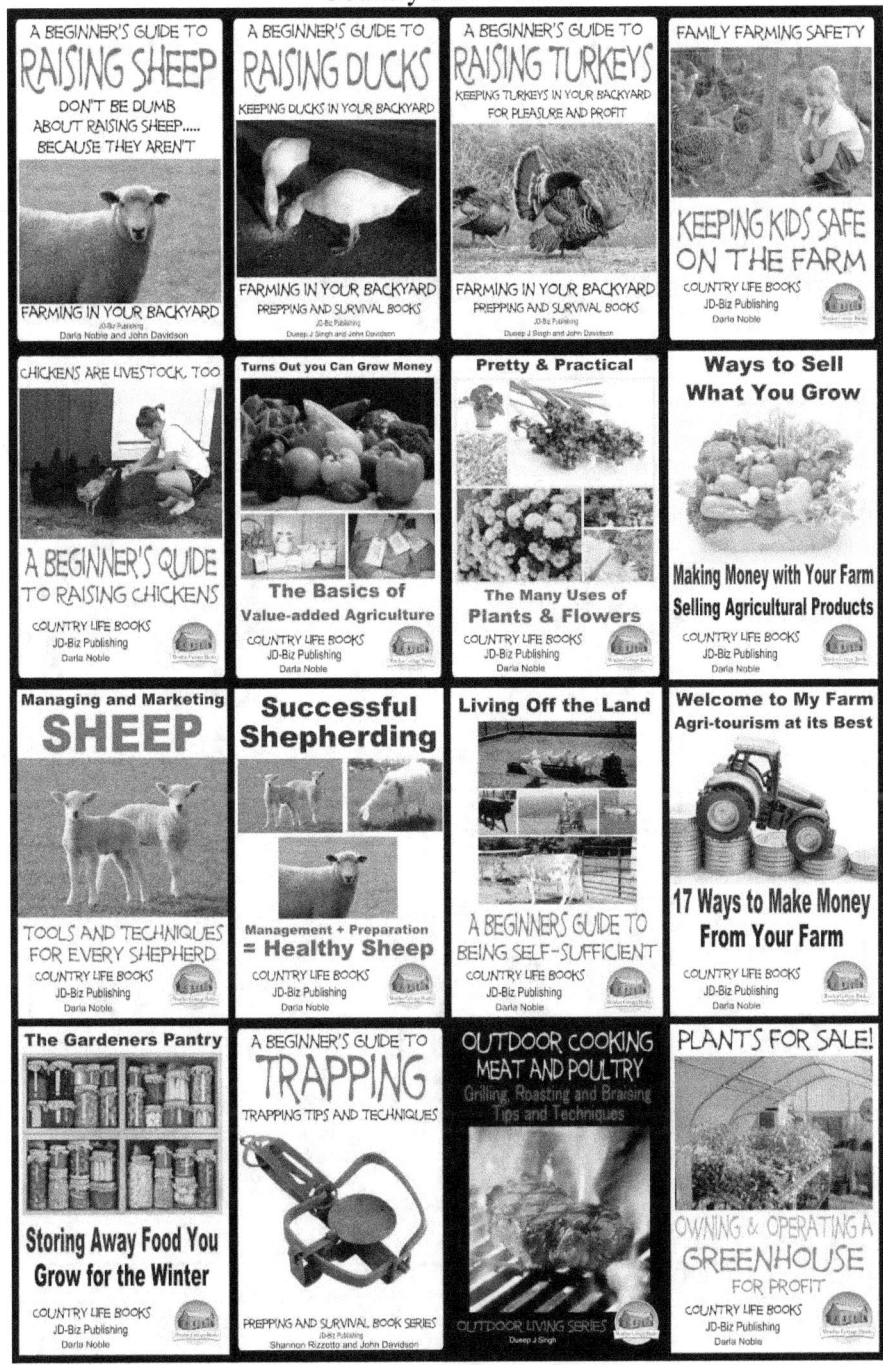

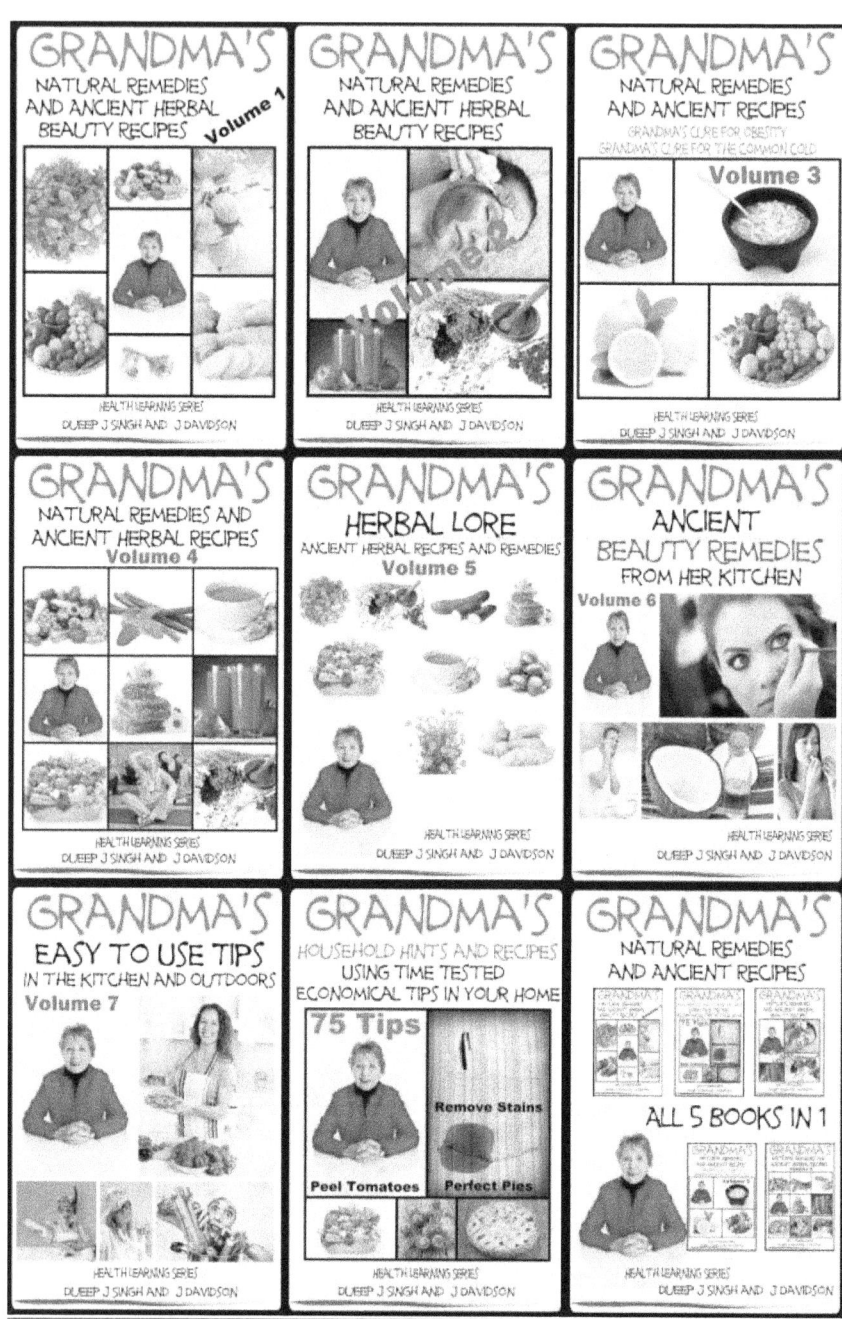

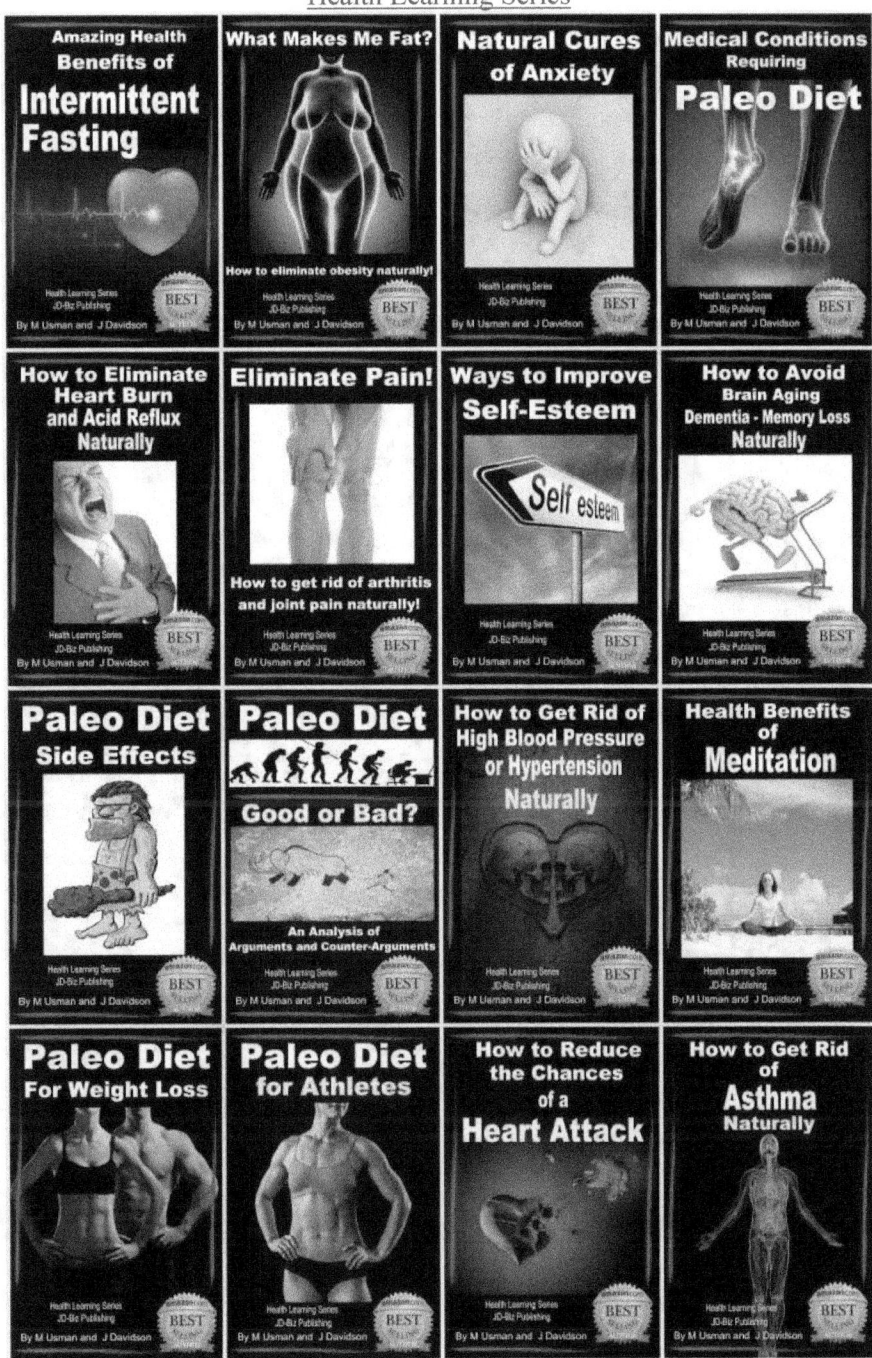

Amazing Animal Book Series

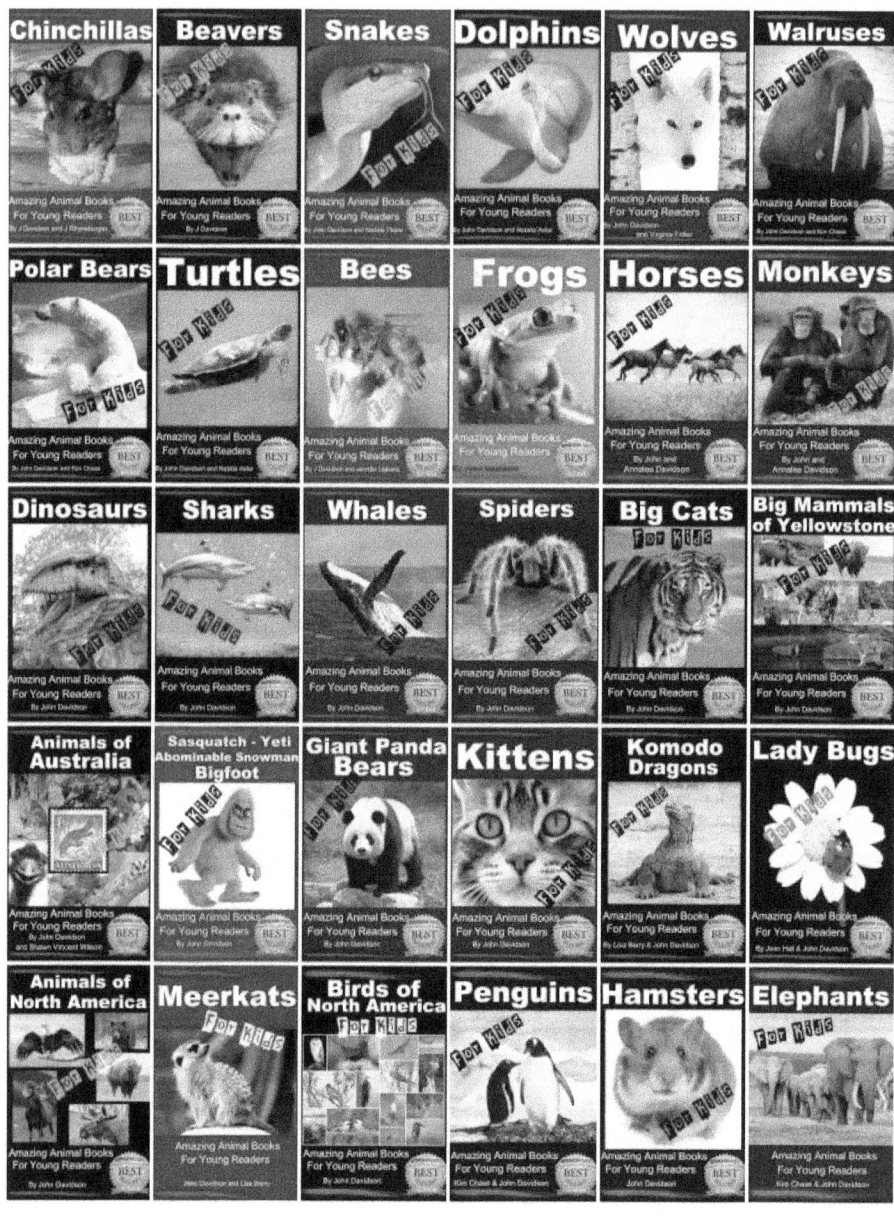

Learn To Draw Series

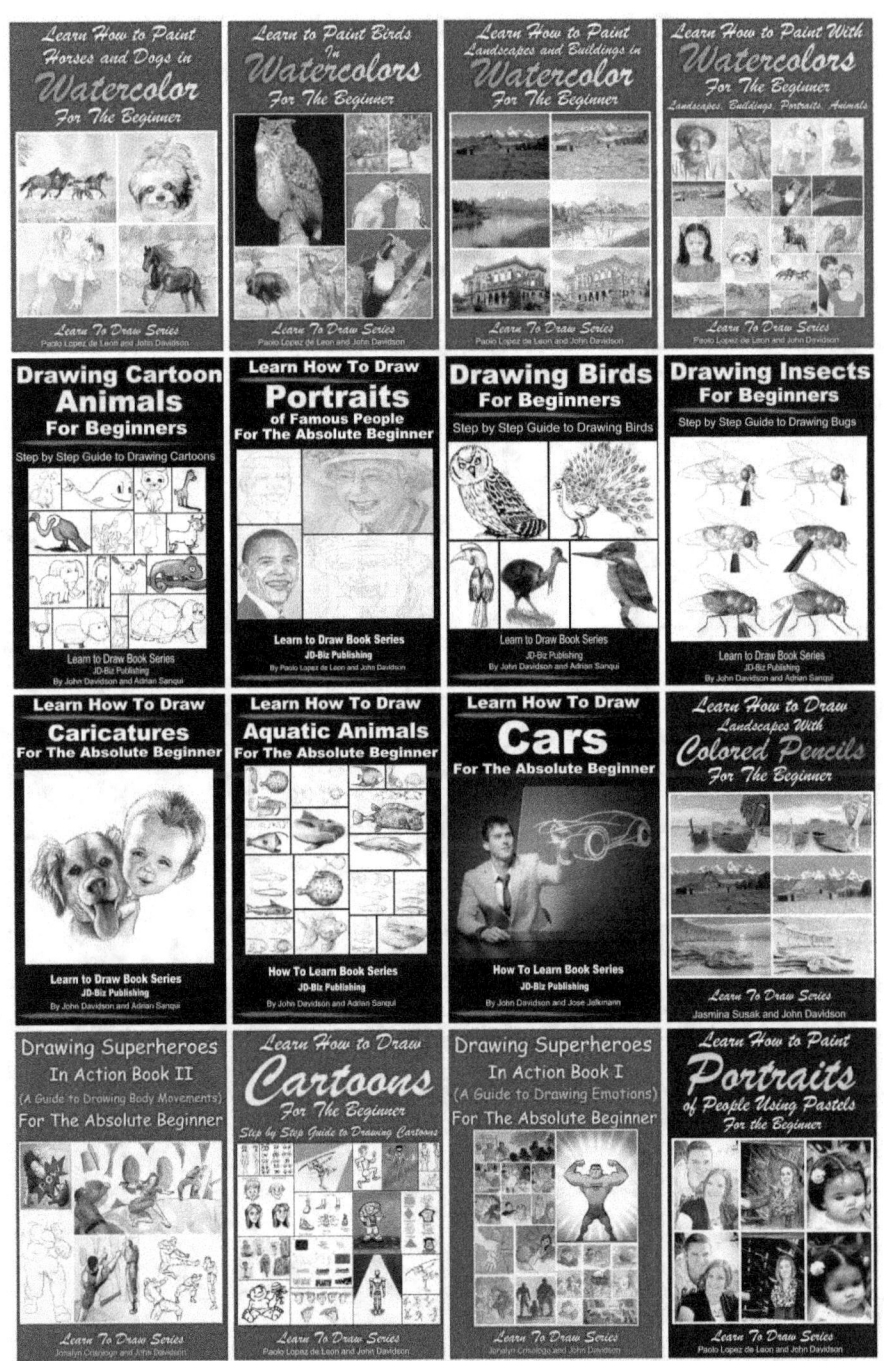

How to Build and Plan Books

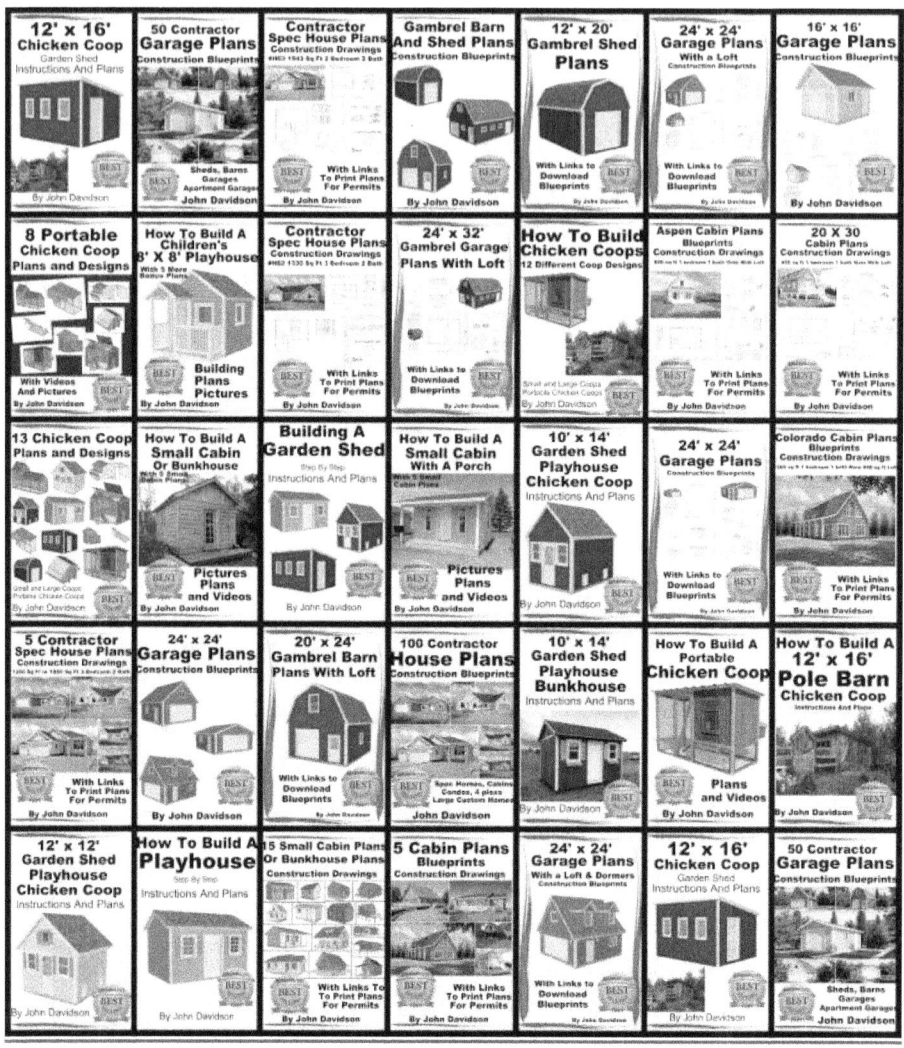

Entrepreneur Book Series

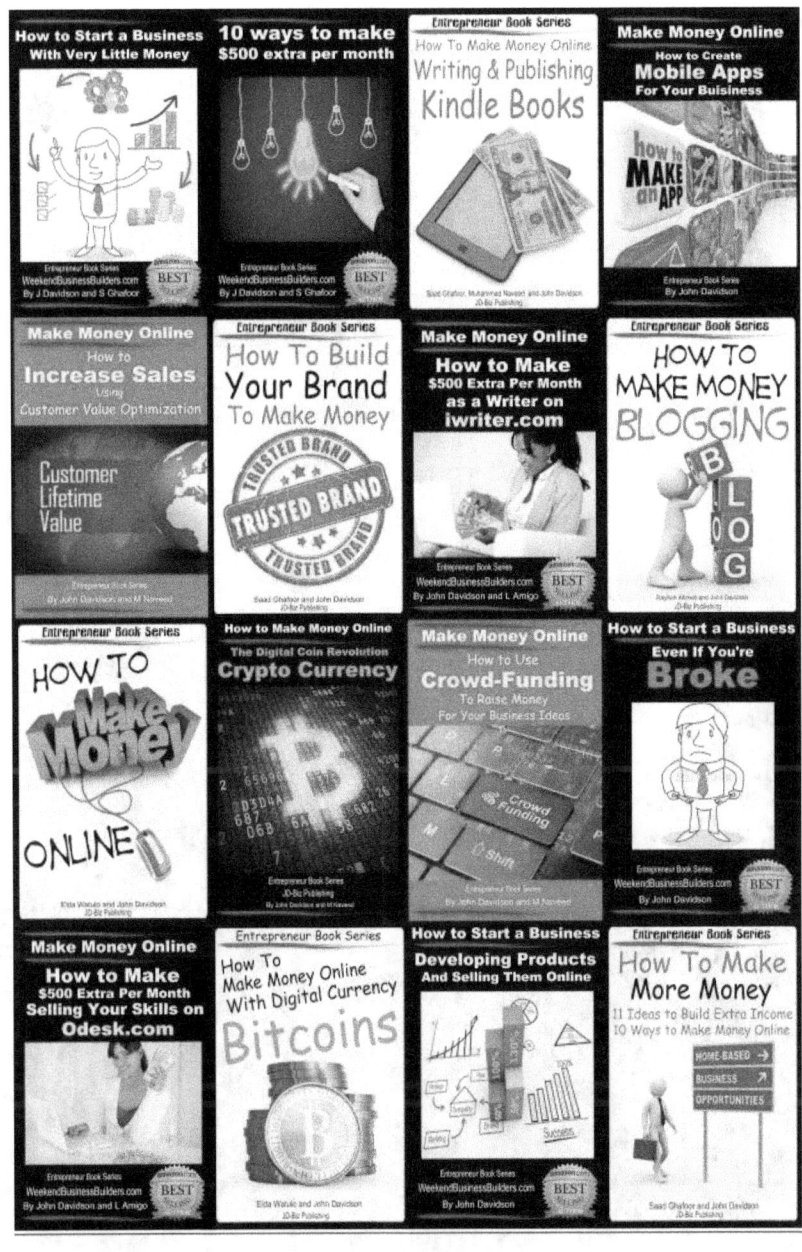

Publisher

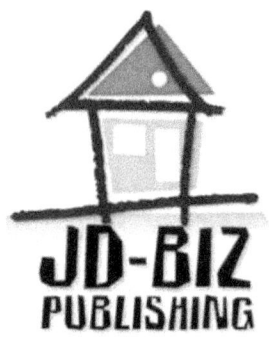

JD-Biz Corp

P O Box 374

Mendon, Utah 84325

http://www.jd-biz.com/

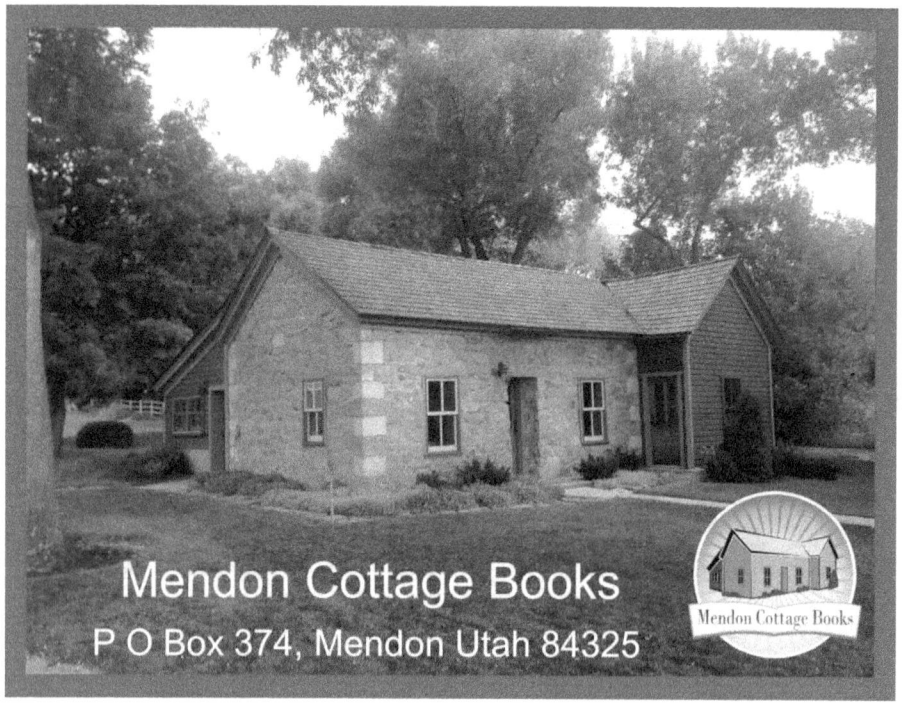

Mendon Cottage Books

P O Box 374, Mendon Utah 84325